DMT

THE DEFINITIVE GUIDE

Zoey Maurice

Chapter One

The definitive guide on how to make dmt

DMT: What Is It?

One class of hallucinogenic drug is DMT. Similar to other hallucinogens, DMT has the ability to change perception. It modifies their perception of environmental stimuli. Substances with psychotic-like effects, such as DMT, are well-known. Of the adverse effects of DMT, paranoia and hallucinations are the most common.

The fact that DMT has been used for centuries distinguishes it from other psychedelic substances available on the market. In contrast to many synthetic medicines, DMT is found in nature. DMT is present in many plants, but the ayahuasca plant is the most well-known source. Having said that, DMT can also be created in a laboratory. Beginning with British chemist Richard Manske in the 1930s, synthetic DMT has been manufactured since then.

In all its synthetic and organic forms, DMT is a prohibited substance even though it occurs naturally. In the 1960s, DMT use for recreational purposes gained popularity. The DEA designated it as a Schedule I drug by the 1970s. Drugs classified as schedule I are the most strictly restricted. Due to its severe negative effects, great potential for misuse, and high likelihood of psychological dependence, DMT was added to the Schedule I list.

DMT is still available on the black market for illegal drugs, according to the DEA, despite being strictly regulated since the 1970s. Purchasing any DMT that is being sold is prohibited. Either DMT is illegally smuggled into the country or synthetic DMT is produced there and brought into the country. The medication can be snorted, smoked, brewed into tea, or taken internally.

Another medication that occurs naturally is marijuana, which is being studied for possible medical uses. In contrast to marijuana, DMT is not recognized to have any medicinal applications. The Food and Drug Administration (FDA) and the Drug Enforcement Administration (DEA) must grant specific approval in order to lawfully purchase DMT for study due to the risks involved.

There is strict regulation of DMT in North America. However, some cultures in South and Central America are still using DMT in religious rituals. Some "guides," both domestically and internationally, lead groups of individuals into the outdoors to administer DMT under their guidance. But since they are not medical experts, using DMT under their supervision is not any safer. Dispelling myths about DMT requires an understanding of both its hazards and how it functions in the body.

Who Takes DMT?

Owing to its illegal status, no organization is able to calculate the number of persons who regularly use DMT. On the basis of US medical and other data, the

Substance Abuse and Mental Health Services Administration (SAMHSA) does, however, create an annual report5 on drug usage. More than 1 million cases of hallucinogenic drug use at some point in the past year are reported by SAMHSA for those over the age of twelve.

Regretfully, there has been an increase in the usage of hallucinogenic drugs for a number of years. Nevertheless, compared to other drug classes, such as stimulants, hallucinogenic drugs do not have nearly as many participants. On the other hand, younger people are using hallucinogenic drugs at a significantly higher rate. The usage of DMT by young people is highly worrying due to its effects and risks.

Individualized treatment plans are offered by Windward Way Recovery to clients of all ages who abuse drugs such as DMT. Helping a loved one get the assistance they require might be greatly aided by our parent and partner guides. Look for a way on how to get a loved one into treatment.

How does DMT appear?

DMT is the hallucinogenic component of the drug ayahuasca

and is present in many different plants.3. Ayahuasca involves boiling a plant that contains DMT and another plant that has a monoamine oxidase inhibitor (MAOI), such harmaline, and then drinking the resulting combination. When manufactured artificially DMT powder is crystalline white in color.

Chapter Two

5-MeO-DMT Succinate Synthesis and Characterization for Clinical Application

A multigram-scale procedure has been created to supply 5-MeO-DMT, a naturally occurring psychedelic substance discovered in the parotid gland secretions of the Incilius alvarius toad, in order to facilitate its clinical application. After a number of synthetic routes were initially investigated, a high-yield optimized Fischer indole reaction to 5-MeO-DMT freebase was chosen as the process. From this, a 1:1 succinate salt was produced, yielding 136 g of crystalline active pharmaceutical ingredient (API) with a net yield of 49% and a peak area of 99.86% by high-performance liquid chromatography (HPLC). In-process monitoring, verified analytical techniques, impurity generation and elimination, and solid-state API characterization—all crucial for later clinical development—are included in the paper.

Overview

Understanding the clinical uses of psychedelic, entactogenic, and dissociative psychoactive drugs like ketamine (5), MDMA (4), LSD (3), psilocybin (1), and DMT (2)— in conjunction with psychotherapy support to promote improved mental health conditions has garnered more attention recently (Figure 1). Research has shown promise in the treatment of anxiety-related illnesses, depression, end-of-life situations, and post-traumatic stress disorder (PTSD) in particular

(1,2).   (1,3–6)   This   study demonstrates   that   certain variables   have   been   linked   to improvements   in   mental   health, even   if   the   therapeutic mechanisms   are   still   poorly understood.   These   variables include   the   potency   of   the mystical   experience   induced   by the   psychedelic,   the   set   and setting of the session, the dosage of   the   drug,   psychological elasticity,   emotional breakthrough,   connectedness, and   increased   neural   entropy. (1,7–10)

Number 1

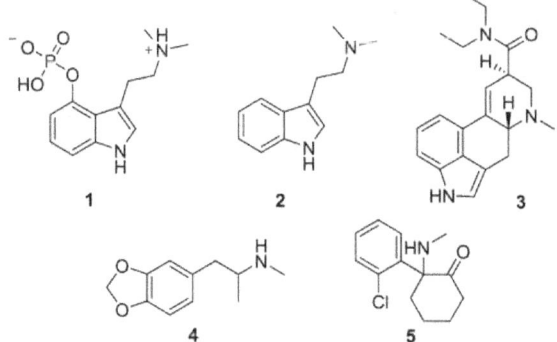

1

2

3

4

5

Step1. List of entactogenic, dissociative, and psychedelic psychoactive substances that have been studied clinically

The main psychoactive ingredient in the parotid gland secretions of the Sonoran Desert toad, Incilius alvarius, is 5-MeO-DMT (6), a naturally occurring tryptamine derivative (Figure 2). (11) It is also known that a number of different plants, bushes, and seeds contain trace amounts of the alkaloid. For at least a century, reports of this substance's psychoactive effects on humans have been documented in the scientific literature. (12–15) Despite historical suggestions that indigenous tribes may have used 5-MeO-DMT, (11) there is no known data to substantiate this claim. Considering that elevated levels of 5-MeO-DMT have recently been found in I. alvarius secretions, its use for spiritual and recreational purposes has reportedly increased. Recent research has revealed that 5-MeO-DMT is present in toad secretion at concentrations of 20–30% of total dry weight, or 200–300 mg of 5-MeO-DMT per dried gram. These values are significantly greater than those found in 5-MeO-DMT obtained from plants (17).

Step 2.

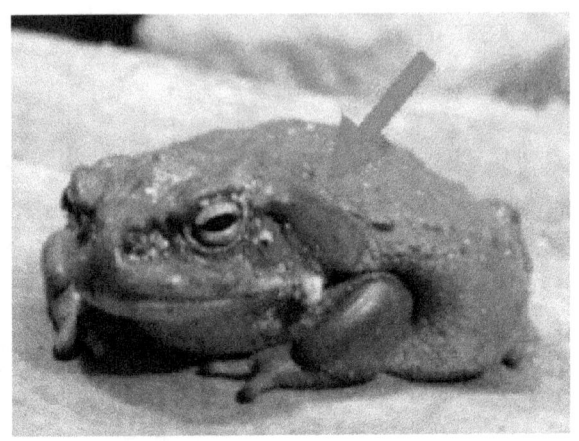

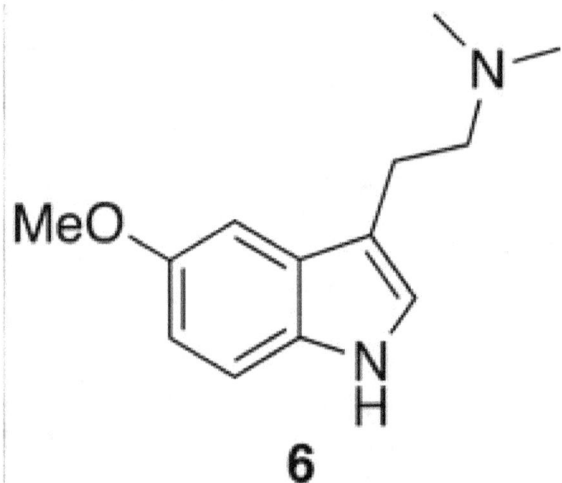

6

Step 2. I (Left). alvarius, with the parotid gland highlighted (photo courtesy of Holger Krisp, Ulm, Germany, 2011 under CC BY 3.0). (Right) 5-MeO-DMT (6) structure

Anecdotal evidence and studies conducted over the past five years indicate that 5-MeO-DMT may be beneficial in the treatment of clinical mental health issues. These results indicate that 5-MeO-DMT (8,9,16–18) causes mystical experiences that are comparable in intensity to those caused by psilocybin, (8) has a much shorter half-life (between 10 and 45 min), depending on the mode of administration, and (19) increases the desired effects when the experience is carefully selected. (20, 21)

A well-established theory states that the primary mechanism underlying frequently experienced psychedelic effects in humans (such as visual hallucinations, altered perceptions of self, time, and space, and unusual thought patterns) is activation of the serotonergic 5-HT2A receptor in the central nervous system (CNS). Notably, in addition to their agonist activity at the 5-HT2A receptor, all currently known psychedelics are also nonselective, simultaneously interacting with a variety of different monoaminergic receptors and transporters in the central nervous system, and as a result, exhibiting varying degrees of synergistic polypharmacology. (22, 23). (24) 5-MeO-DMT has shown sub-micromolar binding affinity for the majority of CNS-expressed serotonin receptor subtypes, with a selectivity of about 300 times for human 5-HT1A (3 ± 0.2 nM) compared to 5-HT2A (907 ± 170 nM) receptor subtypes. (25) Research indicates that 5-HT1A receptor activation may work in concert with 5-HT2A activation to contribute significantly to the subjective and

21

behavioral effects of psychedelics. (26–28) Psilocin, the active metabolite of psilocybin, is approximately five times more selective for human 5-HT2A receptors (107 nM) than 5-HT1A (567 nM), in contrast to 5-MeO-DMT. (29) Coadministration of psilocin with the selective 5-HT1A agonist buspirone, an antianxiety drug, changed the subjective effects of psilocin, substantially lessening the intensity of some visual hallucinations in a controlled trial involving healthy adult volunteers. (30) It's interesting to note that anecdotal reports on 5-MeO-DMT use have often mentioned a lack of the vivid geometric visual hallucinations that are usually connected to other psychedelics. (31)

Currently, there is a lack of a clear knowledge regarding the relationship between the polypharmacology of psychedelics and how it affects their subjective effects. Even though several possible mechanisms, such as enhanced structural plasticity in the prefrontal cortex, have been proposed to explain the therapeutic mode of action of psychedelics, (32) no direct correlation has been found between particular psychedelic pharmacodynamics and beneficial therapeutic outcomes. However, randomized clinical trials including the psychedelic psilocybin (1) continue to show promise in the management of severe mental illnesses such major depressive disorder (MDD). In order to better understand the mode of action of psychedelics in modern controlled clinical research, 5-MeO-DMT appears to be pharmacodynamically distinct from other psychedelics that have been clinically examined.

Psychedelic tryptamines, including DMT (2) and 5-MeO-DMT (6), are not oral active because they undergo fast first-pass metabolism by monoamine oxidase, in contrast to psilocybin. When taken parenterally, they have a much shorter duration of action—typically less than an hour than psilocybin, which has an effect that lasts between five and eight hours. A patient might spend less time in the clinic as a result of the action's shorter duration. Furthermore, it is known that 5-MeO-DMT is 10–20 times more effective in humans than DMT. (13) Compared to other therapeutically researched psychedelics, 5-MeO-DMT has distinct pharmacologic and pharmacokinetic features, including a brief duration of effect and potentially significant 5-HT1A receptor selectivity. These characteristics might be associated with better treatment outcomes in human clinical trials under supervision. In order to investigate this theory, gain a deeper comprehension of the psychotherapeutic effectiveness of 5-MeO-DMT, and facilitate these clinical studies, the active pharmaceutical ingredient (API) must be prepared with sufficient controls to guarantee its identification, potency, purity, and strength. This report focuses on this process's development.

Findings and Discussion

Chapter Three

Choosing the Salt Form and 5-MeO-DMT Dosage

The method of administration that is most frequently described is the vaporization of the freebase medication, which, in comparison to other dosage forms, is usually not a pharmaceutically acceptable strategy. An intramuscular injection has been found to be a better compromise for giving 5-MeO-DMT, even while other alternative modes of administration such dry powder inhalation, transdermal, or intravenous administration are also feasible. Apart from providing accurate dosage metering, intramuscular injection of 5-MeO-DMT in a naturalistic environment has been documented earlier and is said to have a longer duration of effect than other intraperitoneal methods that provide a strong, fast onset. (19) An exact amount of API in the range of 2–15 mg can be delivered by the injectable medication, which is designed as a 20 mg/mL solution of API in sterile water with excipients. This dose range is comparable with the anecdotal reports that have been made with this substance in the past. The 5-MeO-DMT freebase is poorly soluble in water (less than 10 mg/mL), and when exposed to ambient oxygen, the unionized amine may break down and release the equivalent N-oxide degradant (see below). Consequently, a salt form of 5-MeO-DMT that was both pharmaceutically acceptable and soluble in water was needed.

A variety of pharmaceutically acceptable salt forms, including the counterions chloride, sulfate, fumarate, succinate, maleate, lysate, oxalate, benzoate, tartrate, mesylate, or acetate, were taken into consideration from acids with sufficient pKa difference to fully protonate 6.

This research was conducted in tandem with the investigation of feasible synthetic routes to 5-MeO-DMT freebase. (35) The hydrochloride, sulfate, fumarate, and succinate salts were first assessed using analytically pure 5-MeO-DMT freebase. When attempts to produce the sulfate salt resulted in an unmanageable gum, the strategy was dropped. Although the hydrochloride salt was easily made into an apparent crystalline solid, it was discovered that the substance was hygroscopic and deliquescent in high humidity. The salts fumarate and succinate both produced stable, freely-flowing, crystalline solids and were easily manufactured. Because they are easily synthesized, fumarate salts of structurally similar tryptamines are frequently reported. For instance, 36 DMT (2) fumarate has been administered intravenously in clinical trials in the past. (37) Nevertheless, fumaric acid is a recognized Michael acceptor and, in moderate circumstances, has been demonstrated to create covalent compounds with APIs containing amines. As sterile solutions of the 5-MeO-DMT medicinal product may need to be prepared in the future, autoclave sterilization may be necessary.

(38,39) The possibility of this recognized reaction with fumaric acid disqualified it as a suitable salt form. Succinic acid is a dicarboxylic acid with a similar structure to fumaric acid, but it does not have the conjugated double bond and does not react chemically in the same way.

Therefore, more research was done on the succinate salt as a possible salt form that may be approved by pharmaceuticals. The material was prepared and thoroughly characterized in the solid state using techniques such as optical microscopy, 1H nuclear magnetic resonance (NMR), thermogravimetric analysis (TGA), X-ray powder diffraction (XRPD), differential scanning calorimetry (DSC), hyper-DSC, dynamic vapor sorption (DVS), and thermogravimetric analysis (TGA) (see the Supporting Information). In summary, XRPD revealed that most crystallization settings produced a common stable crystalline anhydrate (form A) and that only a small number of conditions resulted in the production of distinct solvated forms for 5-MeO-DMT succinate (1:1), which was not hygroscopic (see the Supporting Information). The results validated 5-MeO-DMT succinate (1:1) as a stable and approved salt form for usage in pharmaceuticals. This salt form was chosen for further study due to its good solid-state characteristics and ease of synthesis.

Chapter Four

Route Scouting for 5-MeO DMT

The ideal synthetic route to 5-MeO-DMT for clinical development would make use of commercially available starting materials, be scalable to easily produce the product in the range of 0.1–1 kg, not rely on fractionation or flash silica gel chromatography, and produce a high-purity final product by using a validated high-performance liquid chromatography (HPLC) method that does not contain any unidentified individual impurities >0.15% peak area. Three potentially workable synthetic pathways were identified by the literature review, and each was investigated and assessed to see if it could satisfy the aforementioned requirements.

Path 1: A reductive amination reaction between formaldehyde and commercially available 5-methoxy tryptamine (7), with sodium cyanoborohydride acting as the reducing agent, was utilized in a seemingly appealing one-step procedure (Scheme 1). (40) Initially, a number of small-scale experiments were assessed using liquid chromatography-mass spectrometry (LCMS) for reaction monitoring. Even though the product was clearly being formed, there were problems with the response that would probably arise again on a greater scale. It was difficult to suppress the Pictet-Spengler reaction to the equivalent tryptoline (8), and it was also difficult to remove this structurally identical and potentially physiologically active byproduct. Although there may be room for improvement with Route 1, it was eventually decided not to pursue further development of the response. A comparable reaction using the N-methylation of tryptamine 7 by methyl iodide has also been proposed; however, this strategy was not taken into consideration for large-scale synthesis because it would unavoidably result in difficult-to-control quaternization at the amine.

Plan 1

Plan1: The Pictet-Spengler Byproduct Formation Mechanism and the Eschweiler-Clarke Reaction to 6

Path 2: The most widely used general procedure for making substituted psychedelic tryptamines is the Speeter–Anthony tryptamine synthesis (Scheme 2), which has also been used to make 5-MeO-DMT in the past. (31,41) The approach was taken into consideration for the large-scale synthesis of 6 from 5-methoxyindole 9 due to recent insights and optimizations from the large-scale synthesis of psilocin and psilocybin produced using an analogous process. (42–44) Using pyrophoric lithium aluminum hydride (LAH) for the final reduction of ketoamide 10 is a crucial step in this process, as is the laborious extraction from solid aluminum waste salts after quenching; the complexity of this procedure tends to rise with scale. According to our results, the reduction stage of tryptamine synthesis typically stalls after 90% conversion, leaving 5–10% of a predicted β-hydroxy intermediate, such 11, remained (Scheme 2). As the crude freebase is worked up, additional adjustments, particularly in an acidic environment, may cause the β-hydroxy impurity to convert into a reactive electrophile, like 12 (Scheme 2), and produce mixes of isomeric dimerized impurities. In order to synthesize

DMT (2) through a mechanism similar to the one shown in Scheme 2, Crookes et al. conducted a comprehensive examination of the creation of comparable dimeric byproducts in the LAH reduction. (45) While Route 2 was a workable procedure, more process development would be necessary to guarantee that the finished product could consistently fulfill high-purity requirements without the need for column chromatography, considering the known difficulties associated with scale-up. Thus, a one-step process based on the Fischer indole reaction was investigated after that.

Plan 2

Plan 2: Synthesis of Speeter-Anthony Tryptaminc and Its Byproducts through Reactive Impurity 11

Plan 3: The development of a scalable process was drawn to the Fischer indole reaction approach to 6 from 4-

methoxyphenylhydrazine (13) and 4,4-diethoxy-N,N-dimethylbutan-1-amine (14), a masked aldehyde protected as the diethyl acetal derivative (Scheme 3A). This approach has several advantages, including a single step of transformation, no requirement for high temperatures, aqueous solvent, and the absence of pyrophoric or air-sensitive reactants like lithium aluminum hydride. Furthermore, prior research has documented its application in the synthesis of 5-MeO-DMT and related substituted N,N-dimethyltryptamines (46). Similarly, comparable procedures have been used in the industry to produce structurally comparable 5-substituted dimethyltryptamine antimigraine medications, including sumatriptan (15), zolmitriptan (16), and rizatriptan (17) (Scheme 3B). Crucially, tryptamines 15–17's medicinal significance offered some reassurance that the crucial butanamine starting material 14—which was used in all three processes—was well-characterized and would continue to be widely accessible at a reasonable price.

Path 3

A - Fischer Indole (FI) reaction

13 + **14** → Brønsted or Lewis acids → **6**

B - Commercially available dimethyltryptamine (synthesized *via* the FI route)

15 **16** **17**

Plan 3: (A) The Fischer Indole Reaction was used to prepare six, and (B) the Analogous Process was used to prepare approved antimigraine medications

The reaction was first carried out in refluxing dilute aqueous sulfuric acid solution in accordance with the previously reported technique (Table 1, entry 1). (46) Phenylhydrazine,

46

the limiting reagent, was consumed in less than two hours, according to reaction monitoring by LCMS. The crude reaction purity was around 63% peak area, with various high-molecular-weight contaminants accounting for the remaining 37% peak area. Chromatography would have probably been necessary for the process to isolate the product with a high enough level of purity due to the substantial impurity profile. By coincidence, we saw that an aliquoted LCMS sample that had been removed before reflux and had been prepared in acetonitrile rather than water had almost completely completed the reaction at ambient temperature or lower, containing virtually solely 6 and very few byproducts. In response to this finding, a follow-up experiment was conducted at room temperature over the course of an overnight period, employing a 1:1 water/acetonitrile solvent mixture to verify an 88% conversion to the product by LCMS (Table 1, entry 2). The procedure was carried out again and further circumstances were investigated in light of the positive outcomes.

Chapter Five

Conditions for Reaction Optimization

Separated yield

With acetonitrile as the cosolvent, the reaction was observed to finish in 3 hours when the temperature was raised to 40 °C (Table 1, entry 3). Several additional reactions were tested with various cosolvents, such as methanol, dimethyl sulfoxide (DMSO), 2-methyltetrahydrofuran

(2-MeTHF), and dichloromethane (DCM) (Table 1, entries 4–7), in comparison to the same volume of water under otherwise identical conditions (Table 1, entry 8), in order to better understand the role of the cosolvent. All of the cosolvents that were tested were shown to be beneficial in boosting reaction conversion, with the exception of water-miscible polar aprotic DMSO, which produced outcomes that were on par with acetonitrile. Additionally, methanol significantly improved the reaction. Additionally, the water-immiscible solvents DCM and 2-MeTHF somewhat increased reaction conversion.

According to these results, the majority of cosolvents enhanced the reaction's conversion and purity profile, and the water-miscible polar aprotic cosolvents significantly accelerated the rate of synthesis of 6 while reducing side reactions. Even while reactants 13 and 14 seemed to be water soluble when the cosolvent was not present, we reasoned that it might have helped to dissolve one of the reactants or stopped the development of hydrophobic clusters. The discovery that the majority of side reaction impurities generated in the absence of a cosolvent were suggestive of high-molecular-weight oligomers, which might develop from localized high-concentration clusters of beginning reactants, lends support to the idea. Even while acetonitrile and DMSO behaved similarly, acetonitrile was chosen for continued research because DMSO's low volatility and high boiling point could have added more complexity, which is why it was eventually removed from the workup.

Diethyl acetal 14 might be lowered to 1.05 equiv in relation to limiting reagent 13 according to additional optimization.

Without observable effects on the crude reaction profile or reaction rate, the acetonitrile cosolvent was lowered from 10 to 5 volumes and the temperature was lowered to 35 °C (Table 1, entry 9). Moreover, the reaction profile was barely affected by stressing the same reaction for an additional 28 hours, resulting in a 1% decrease in the crude reaction mixture's HPLC purity (Table 1, entry 9b). Advantageously, the reaction showed no ill effects from prolonged hold times, indicating that reaction time was not a crucial process parameter and that, when the process was performed at scale, considerable temporal flexibility could be possible. The process was scaled to 100 mmol (about 35 g) based on the improvements mentioned, and isolation conditions were investigated to finally produce high-purity 6 as the succinate salt in 80% isolated yield (Table 1, entry 9).

Chapter Six

Optimizing Isolation, Workup, and Salt Formation

Solution

Using dichloromethane as an extraction solvent for the freebase after basification and as a washing solvent for the acidic crude reaction mixture, the crude freebase product was first separated using a standard acid/base workup technique. A heavy insoluble oil impurity was found to develop in larger-scale reactions requiring prolonged hold periods of the freebase product in methylene chloride. It was anticipated that (48–52) 5-

MeO-DMT underwent a similar reaction to create the quaternary ammonium byproduct 18, which is in line with other published studies on the chemical reactivity of DMT and other tertiary amines with methylene chloride (Scheme 4). The identity of structure 18 (Scheme 4 and Supporting Information S14) was supported by the 1H NMR analysis of the crude heavy oil, which yielded a singlet at 5.69 ppm that integrated to 2H. Product 6's apparent reactivity with dichloromethane suggested that a different solvent be used during the workup procedure, particularly at bigger scales where longer hold times could be necessary.

Plan 4

Plan 4: Formation of Degradant 18 for the Suspected Dichloromethane Adduct Annotated with a 1H NMR Shift

In biphasic aqueous workups, 2-Methyltetrahydrofuran (2-MeTHF) has been proposed as a good dichloromethane alternative in the past. (53) We discovered that

2-MeTHF formed a clean phase split with the acidic aqueous crude reaction mixture, negating the requirement to distill the acetonitrile cosolvent. Freebase 6 was also shown to be extremely soluble. Furthermore, because 2-MeTHF is manufactured industrially using biorenewable techniques, it is a greener solvent choice for process chemistry. The acetonitrile cosolvent was distilled before workup on a lesser scale. On a bigger scale, the workup went straight into a liquid-liquid washing stage, skipping this distillation altogether. Data from later steps would suggest that some product was lost during the initial washing stage as it was removed into the organic phase. This could be attributable to enhanced partitioning brought on by the presence of acetonitrile.

Chapter Seven

Purification at Freebase

Using LC-UV high-resolution mass spectrometry (HRMS) to analyze the crude freebase extract, it was discovered that the crude reaction mixture contained many isomeric dimer-like products, which together accounted for around 8% of the total peak area. Different attachment locations (denoted by red circles) for the dimer are also plausible, but HRMS analysis provided m/z 534.3803 with MS/MS fragmentation to m/z 316.2383 for each of the isomers, corroborating the putative structure 19 (Scheme 5 and corroborating Information S15). For the isometric impurity corresponding to m/z 534.3803, the HRMS results validated the identify of a triamine regardless of connection. Even though it was first discovered that ethanol was a good solvent for recrystallizing the succinate salt of 6, it was later discovered that the isomeric dimers co-crystallized with 6 at quantities above the limits for impurities. As an alternative, we hypothesized that there would be a notable difference in retention between triamine isomers of 19 and monoamine 6 on silica gel, allowing for the removal of polar contaminants through filtration through a tiny silica plug while still enabling the product 6 to elute easily. Ten percent methanol in acetone was found to provide such separation in mobile phase screening experiments using thin-layer chromatography; polar dimer impurities remained adhered to the baseline and the product spot for number six migrated with a retention factor (Rf) of approximately 0.3 (Supporting Information S16). Dichloromethane is frequently employed in separations with polar amines, however given the reactivity difficulties mentioned above, it was deemed undesirable. Methanol/acetone is an uncommon eluent with silica gel. In the preparative stage, 80–90% mass of the input crude freebase could be recovered by filtering through a 5% silica pad and washing the pad with 100 vol of 10% methanol in acetone. The polar dimeric impurities, on the other hand, remained attached to the baseline and were successfully eliminated.

Plan 5

19
Exact Mass: 534.3803

20
Exact Mass: 316.2383

Plan 5: Alleged Dimer Impurity Configuration and MS/MS Fragmentation

The red circles represent different attachment locations.

In the HPLC analysis of the resultant eluent after the silica filtration stage, a hitherto unseen degradant was detected in up to 3% of the peak area. Oxidation degradant 21, the N-oxide of 6, was definitively identified as the degradant. The structure was first confirmed by HRMS (Supporting Information S17), and it was then definitively described 21 by chemical synthesis and further 1H and 13C NMR characterization (Scheme 6 and Supporting Information S18 and S19). Since N-oxide 21 is a metabolite of 6 (54) according to prior in vitro and in vivo metabolism research, there would be some leeway in the amount of this degradant that can be present in the API.

Plan 6

Plan 6: Creation of N-Oxide 21 Formation of Succinate Salt

The succinic acid salt of 6 was easily isolated using smaller-scale development procedures. Simply add 1 equiv of succinic acid to a solution of freebase 6 in acetone, then filter the resulting insoluble crystalline precipitate. Subsequently, we discovered that adding an activated charcoal washing step reduced the small color variations we saw in the isolated end product. The usage of several commercial sources of phenylhydrazine 13 was shown to be associated with color variation, despite the fact that all lots were tested to >98% purity upon arrival. To create the succinate salt in a methanol solution at a volume that did not originally cause precipitation, the process was changed. Activated charcoal was added to the resultant mixture, which was filtered and then concentrated. To produce a crystalline solid that was consistent with the intended polymorphic form, the resultant solid succinate salt was slurried in acetone, filtered, and dried. A net yield of 49% was obtained from the method, yielding 136 g of isolated succinic acid salt of 6 with a peak area of 99.86% HPLC purity. At 0.14% peak area, the N-oxide degradant 21 was the only contaminant that could be detected. After salt production, it was discovered that ethanol worked well as a re-crystallization solvent for additional purification of the succinate salt of 6, if needed. This was not mentioned in the larger-scale synthesis, but it was nevertheless found to meet the requisite purity requirements.

Chapter Eight

Prospective Optimization

The Fischer indole reaction to six easily supplied API complied with all requirements. The primary goal was to produce a high-purity product; however, additional optimization can raise the yield without lowering the quality of the finished product. Product conversion was as high as 90%, according to HPLC data, however isolated freebase recovery was only 57%. Furthermore, an isolated yield of 80% was obtained in the smaller-scale development reaction (Table 1, entry 9). The primary distinction between the two procedures was the cosolvent's distillation before workup and the significant yield loss that happened during the first liquid-liquid washing stage, wherein 10–20% of the product was recovered from the first wash's acidic aqueous layer. To make up for this loss, the washes might one day be back-extracted. It would be ideal to do away with the silica pad filtration step when scaling up even more. When separating the freebase product from high-MW dimers like 19, vacuum distillation of the crude freebase may be a suitable substitute. While re-crystallization techniques could not effectively remove dimer contaminants from succinate salt, it may be possible to avoid silica pad filtering by investigating the re-crystallization of other salt forms before succinate salt is generated. Further tuning of the reaction conditions could be investigated as an alternative to purification techniques in order to increase the reaction's selectivity toward the synthesis of 6 and reduce side reactions.

Section of Experiments

Typical Experimental Procedures

Solvents and raw materials acquired commercially were used

in the reactions. All commercially acquired reagents were used as received after identity testing, unless specified otherwise. Temperature control was achieved using a Julabo FPW91-SL Ultra-Low Refrigerated-Heating circulator in a 5 L Borosilicate Glass 3.3 jacketed glass reactor during the reactions. A Buchi Rotavapor R-220 Pro was used for distillations larger than five liters. Thin-layer chromatography (TLC) was used to monitor the reactions using EMD/Merck silica gel 60 F254-precoated plates (0.25 mm). Using a CombiFlash Rf system (Teledyne ISCO Inc.), prefabricated RediSepRf columns were used for flash column chromatography. Bruker Avance 400 and Avance 500 NMR spectra were obtained at 400 and 101 MHz, respectively, and 500 and 126 MHz, respectively. Using a Waters HSS T3 column (2.5 μm, 2.1 mm × 30 mm) run in gradient mode with H_2O (0.1% formic acid) and acetonitrile (0.1% formic acid) mobile phases at 0.6 mL/min, process development and reaction monitoring were carried out using a Waters Acquity I-Class UPLC. A volume of 0.1 μL was injected after the samples had been diluted to around 1 mg/mL in either acetonitrile or water. A diode array detector picked up chromatographic peaks at 269 nm. In ESI-positive mode, high-resolution mass spectra were obtained in line with UV using a Waters Xevo G2-XS QTof. Using a Waters MSe experiment, low and high collision energy mass spectra were collected.

2-N,N-dimethylethanamine 6-(5-Methoxy-1H-indol-3-yl)

4-methoxyphenylhydrazine hydrochloride (145.0 g; 0.83 mol, 1.0 equiv, purity >98% verified by HPLC) was charged into a dry, clean, 5-liter reactor. Water (1.45 L, 10 vol) was then added, and the mixture was kept at 20–25 degrees Celsius in a nitrogen environment. After that, the reactor's contents were agitated at 30 to 35 °C, and a dark crimson suspension was seen. Concentrated H_2SO_4 (47.7 mL, 0.91 mol, 1.1 equiv) was carefully added to the suspension dropwise over the course of 10 minutes under a nitrogen environment, keeping the temperature below 40 °C. The brown/red solution was heated to 35–40 °C (with a target temperature of 37 °C) and agitated for a further 10 minutes (note that this addition is slightly exothermic). At a temperature of between 35 and 40 °C, a solution of 4,4-diethoxy-N,N-dimethylbutan-1-amine (14) (165.0 g, 0.87 mol, 1.05 equiv) was produced in acetonitrile (0.58 L, 4.0 vol) and introduced dropwise to the reactor under a nitrogen environment over approximately 60 min. After rinsing with 145 mL of 1.0 vol of acetonitrile, the addition funnel was dropped dropwise into the reactor. For an extra four hours, the contents were shaken and the temperature was kept at 40 °C. For HPLC analysis and reaction completion, a sample of the reaction mixture was aliquoted with a target limit of ≤2% peak area for the limiting reagent.

(Outcome: 4-Methoxyphenylhydrazine: 1.86% areas) The mixture's contents were moved to a 10 L reactor after it was cooled to 20–25 °C. 2-MeTHF was used to wash the acidic aqueous solution (2 × 2.03 L, 14.0 vol). The layers were given fifteen minutes to settle after each wash. The upper 2-MeTHF wash was disposed of, while the lower acidic aqueous layer was recovered. After replenishing the acidic aqueous layer in the reactor, a dropwise addition of sodium hydroxide solution (4 M, 0.65 L, 4.5 vol) was made while the temperature was kept at 20–25 °C. This brought the pH to 11–12, resulting in a milky suspension. 2-MeTHF (3 × 1.45 L, 10.0 vol) was used to extract the suspension; after each extraction, the layers were allowed to settle for fifteen minutes, after which the upper organic layer was collected and the lower alkaline water layer was separated into a drum. After discarding the lower aqueous layer, the mixed organic layers of 2-MeTHF were moved to a 20 L flask. Vacuo was used to concentrate the solution into an oily, amber residue. By dissolving the residue again and using new 2-MeTHF (1.45 L, 10 vol), residual water was eliminated azeotropically. The concentration stage was then repeated. After one hour at 40–45°C and vacuum (10–20 mbar), this oily residue was dried on a rotatory evaporator to produce 117.68 g (or 64.9% theoretical yield) of crude 5-MeO-DMT freebase After dissolving the crude freebase in 1.45 L of 10.0 vol of acetone, the mixture was passed through a silica pad (230–400 mesh, 725 g, 5 wt). Acetone/MeOH (9:1, v-v, 14.5 L, 100.0 vol) was used to elute the pad. The mixed filtrates were concentrated to produce a pale clear orange oil that slowly solidified on standing, yielding 102.94 g of pure 5-McO-DMT freebase (56.8% yield, 98.27% area by HPLC).

In conclusion

In order to facilitate first-in-human clinical trials, the first production cycle produced enough API to address current clinical and nonclinical needs with 6. An enhanced Fischer indole reaction with the beneficial addition of acetonitrile cosolvent to produce crude freebase 6 was one of the developed process's main characteristics. The workup included a silica pad filtration for an intermediate purification step, utilizing greener solvent options. Then, using methanol and an activated charcoal decolorizing step, the 1:1 succinic acid salt was made. The last purification process was using an acetone slurry. The equivalent N-oxide 21, a minor API degradation product, was discovered, created, and studied. A total of 49% of the final product was extracted, yielding 136 g of API with 99.86% HPLC purity. The established process's intrinsic controllability and scalability will guarantee that the clinical demands for 6 are fulfilled both now and in the future.

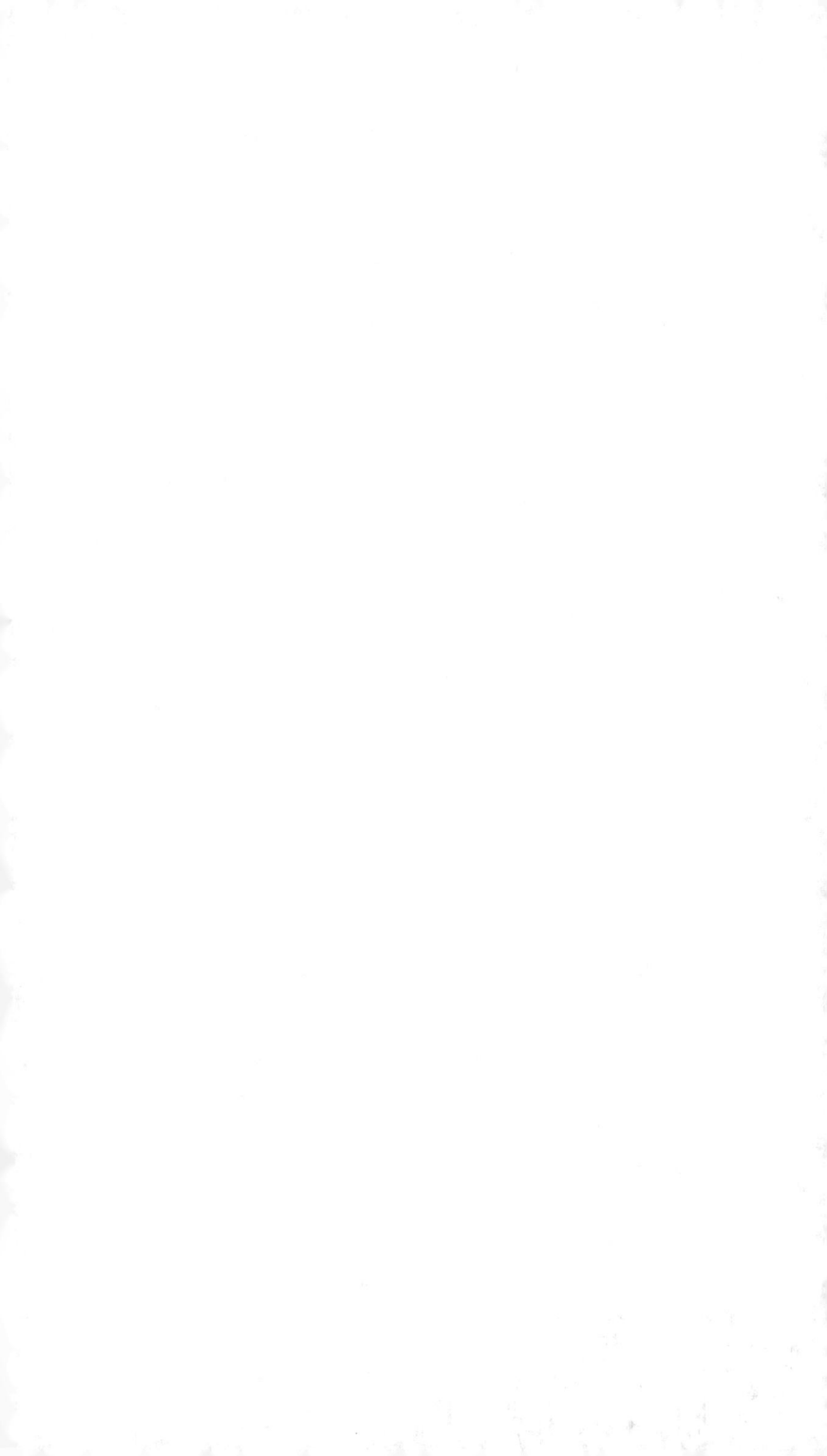